American Medical Association
Physicians dedicated to the health of America

The Physician in Transition: *Managing the Job Interview*

Donald L. Double

© 1997, American Medical Association

Order information:
Additional copies of
The Physician in Transition: Managing the Job Interview
may be obtained from the American Medical Association
for $14.95 AMA members and $19.95 non-members.
For order information, please call 800 621-8335.
Ask for product # OP 206297.

For more information on career management,
be sure to visit the AMA Web site at
http://www.ama-assn.org

ISBN: 89970-849-8

BP37.96-743.3M.12/96

Contents

Acknowledgments 4
Introduction 5
Preparing for the Interview 8
20 Crucial Questions 15
Setting the Stage 23
Running the Gauntlet 28
Special Situations 33
A Final Word 35

Acknowledgments

Donald L. Double, author, is executive vice president of Redirections, Inc, a Chicago firm that provides executive assessment and coaching services to Fortune 100 companies. He has spent the last two decades assessing and coaching senior executives. In health care, he has worked for the former Baxter Travenol, creating and delivering management development programs, and in human resources for the Rehabilitation Institute, Chicago. A consultant for the past 16 years, he has worked extensively for health care organizations, including the American Medical Association, American Hospital Association, and University of Illinois Hospital and Clinics, providing assistance in executive assessment, coaching and team building, and downsizing. In this last capacity, he has assisted hundreds of executives in making career transitions.

Malinda D. Hale, CMSR, principal at Physician Options, Inc, Kingwood, Texas, and Carol E. Sprague, senior recruiter at the American Medical Association, Chicago, provided additional insights.

Editorial support for this publication was provided by Sharyn Sweeney Bills. Product development was managed by Suzanne Fraker, senior acquisition editor, Book and Product Group, at the American Medical Association.

Introduction

The Interview—Why It's Important

Like most physicians, you probably prepared for your professional life by focusing exclusively on acquiring the scientific skills you needed to render the best possible medical care to patients. Now, however, you're faced with a different challenge. As your career experiences the impact of the revolution in health care that is so dramatically changing medical practice today, a rude awakening may occur.

Once upon a time, physicians could simply hang out a shingle and wait for their careers to happen. Today, opportunities and options abound. You may choose to align yourself with a medical group, join a managed care organization, go to work for a health maintenance organization, seek capital backing for an entrepreneurial venture, or find a place to apply your professional skills in an administrative or managerial capacity within a corporate structure.

Most of these options will require you to pass a test your medical education never prepared you for—undergoing an interview. When you do, you'll be judged on more than competence in your basic professional skills. In a matter of no more than minutes, someone will make a highly subjective judgment about you. In that short time, you'll be either accepted or found wanting, and the final decision may have only a little to do with your actual qualifications for the position in question.

> **You'll be judged on more than competence in your basic professional skills.**

Stories about the irrationality of the interview process abound. One prominent businessperson, it's been said, made employment decisions on the basis of whether candidates interviewed at lunch salted their food before tasting it, the rationale being that those who did so acted out of habit rather than judgment. Apocryphal? Perhaps. But the point of the story is indisputable. The outcome of most interviews is the result of intuitive reactions or feelings that often cannot be explained, even by the interviewers.

Does that mean that there is nothing you can do to influence the outcome of an interview? Not at all. You may not be able to guarantee the outcome of an interview, but by understanding the process and systematically preparing yourself for it, you can change the balance so that the weight of probable positive reaction rests on your side.

A Two-Part Challenge

In undergoing an interview, there's more at stake than just winning the approval of the interviewer, of course. In focusing on the interview solely as a challenge to accomplish that objective, many interviewees lose sight of an important fact. Interviewing successfully means not only earning the approval of the interviewer, but achieving an equally important goal: determining whether the opportunity that's presented is the right one for you. It's a two-part process by which not only the candidate but the opportunity itself should be put to the test. Of what value is it, after all, to achieve a position that's not the right one for you?

The interview, therefore, should be viewed not as an obstacle course to be run, but as an opportunity—an opportunity to present yourself in the best light and to gather as much information about the position and the organization as you share about yourself.

The Anatomy of an Interview

What is an interview? Writing in a 1994 issue of the *Journal of Applied Psychology,* Michael A. McDaniel and coauthors described the interview as "... a selection procedure designed to predict future job performance on the basis of applicants' oral responses to oral inquiries." And that is how most interviewers are likely to consciously approach the task.

Toward that end, while examining your education and experience, interviewers are likely to be seeking the answers to these questions, as well:

- What motivates the candidate?
- How does the candidate make decisions?

- How high is the candidate's energy level?
- What is the level of the candidate's self-esteem?
- Why is the candidate interested in this opportunity and this organization?
- What experience can the candidate demonstrate that will help us achieve our goals?
- What technical or professional skills does the candidate have that can contribute to achievement of our goals?
- What value does the candidate place on relationships?
- In what way is the candidate's behavior likely to affect our current team?
- How skilled is the candidate at problem solving?
- What are the candidate's most prominent intellectual skills?
- How does the candidate react under pressure?
- How well will the candidate represent our organization?
- Does the candidate exhibit passion about work and life?
- What interests does the candidate have outside of work that demonstrate maturity, well-roundedness, and the ability to bring to the job perspective and balance from extracurricular activities?

Whatever specific questions are asked in the interview, these are the questions that an interviewer really needs answers to. Let's see how you can prepare to provide them.

Preparing for the Interview

What You Need to Know About the Opportunity

Knowledge is power. The more knowledgeable you are about the organization you're interviewing with, the better prepared you'll be to demonstrate how you can contribute to achievement of its goals and objectives—and the better able to assess whether you want to devote your professional time and energies to doing so.

- What is the principal business of the target organization?
- What organizations dominate its industry? Where does the target organization rank, and what is its reputation?
- What marketplace strategies does it pursue—for example, industry leader? largest provider? most prolific developer of new products?
- What are its key products and/or services?
- What niches within the industry does it pursue?
- Who are its major competitors?
- What major trends have affected the organization during the past 3 years?
- What trends are likely to affect it for the next 3 years?
- What factors are most likely to shape those trends—government regulations? foreign competition? mergers or acquisitions? others?
- What problems are these trends likely to pose for the organization?
- What is its financial condition?
- Who are the organization's leaders? What are their backgrounds and lengths of tenure?

The more knowledgeable you are about the organization you're interviewing with, the better prepared you'll be to demonstrate how you can contribute to achievement of its goals and objectives.

Can you answer those questions? If not, it's time to do some homework, because that's the kind of information you'll need to have at hand to shape intelligent questions and interview responses.

You don't need to become an expert, of course; unless you already have substantial experience in the industry, that's more than is likely to be expected of you at this point in your career. But you do need to know the framework in which the organization operates and be able to demonstrate that you understand the dynamics that affect its performance.

Where to Find What You Need to Know

- So numerous are the medical and business journals in print today that listing them here would be impractical. But your local library should be able to identify journals published for any industry you specify.
- *Forbes, Fortune, The Economist, Business Week,* and the *Harvard Business Review* are among business periodicals that occasionally provide comprehensive reviews of various industries.
- Nexus/Lexus is a business research service that can be accessed via any of the major electronic services, such as America OnLine, or CompuServe. Clippings of articles on any subject can be ordered through such services.
- Dun & Bradstreet reports are available on any organization that has ever borrowed money. These reports may be available through various library or on-line services, as well as through D&B itself—albeit at a relatively high cost.
- The research departments of area newspapers may be able to provide clippings of relevant coverage of local organizations.
- Virtually every major industry supports an association devoted to its interests, some of which may be willing to share their research with you. The *Directory of Associations,* available at most local libraries, provides a comprehensive list.

Much important data on publicly held organizations is also available directly from the organization itself. Call its department of stockholder services and ask for the most recent prospectus, annual report, and K-1 report. The annual report will provide up-to-date information on major products or services and overall trends in growth (or lack thereof), as well as information on important issues facing the organizations and the strategies in place to address them. K-1 reports provide detailed financial data and discuss legal actions in which the organization is involved.

A prospectus, which may have been developed when the organization was started and updated periodically thereafter, may be more or less useful, depending on its timeliness. Even if it is out of date, however, it is likely to provide useful information on the history of the organization and its intended place within the industry. Public relations or public affairs departments may also provide annual reports and other literature on the organization and its products or services.

Organizations that are not publicly held may pose more of a research challenge. Consider checking *Who's Who in American Industry*. And, whatever the organization's ownership, don't forget one of the most valuable resources of all: your own personal contacts within an organization.

If the selection process is going to involve an interview with key organization executives, you'll want to know more about those executives, too. Information that may be useful includes:

- Where they were educated.
- Where they were previously employed.
- When they joined the organization, under what circumstances, and what they are assigned to accomplish there.

What You Need to Know About Yourself

"Tell me about yourself." That's a question you're likely to hear, in one form or another, in virtually every interview encounter. Remember that list of questions on page 6 that outlines those things the interviewer really wants to know about you? What you reveal in responding may tell an interviewer more about what he or she wants to know about you than any other information you exchange. Really understanding who you are and what you want out of life, and analyzing and inventorying your strengths and weaknesses, is an essential—and usually overlooked—step in preparing responses to the questions designed to obtain those insights.

> "Tell me about yourself."

Taking stock of yourself as part of this process has even more important implications, however. The career decisions you make will have a major, long-term impact on your professional and personal life—and, if you have family responsibilities, on the lives of family members, too. Whether you are interested in buying a business, making a career change, or joining a practitioners' group or a managed care organization, it's important to make the best choices possible to fulfill your lifelong goals. You truly need to know yourself to know what's best for you and others you're responsible to. Objectively answering these questions

It's Another World

It may not seem fair, but an important lesson for physicians to learn when they're seeking employment beyond the world of clinical practice is that the attributes that spell success as a physician may be inappropriate or even counterproductive to achievement in the world of business. Here are some transitions you may need to make.

From team leader to team player. Medical education and practice encourage you to take charge. Although accountability is increasingly becoming a given in health care, many physicians still are oriented to individual action or acting as the captains of their own ships. But consensus is the currency of modern business. It's your ability to contribute as a member of a team, and not your leadership skills alone, by which you'll be judged.

From results-oriented to process-oriented. The tasks and goals of medical practice are singular and relatively simple—cure, palliate, or otherwise support the patient. Those of business tend to be far more numerous and complex. While medical practice emphasizes individual action, doing business requires orchestrating a myriad of activities to achieve a given outcome. Each team member's activities must be coordinated with those of many others. Therefore, in the business world, having the patience to participate in the processes of doing business is often as important as the results achieved.

and committing the answers to writing should also help you gain the insight you need to make wise choices.

- What theme or themes underlie your life? Review the choices you've made at major milestones in your life. What are the factors, such as childhood and school experiences or the influence of others, that have been driving you? Consciously or unconsciously, those choices probably have been consistent with long-term drives toward certain goals. Typically, there is a thread, a theme, or a striving in a consistent direction that underlies all our lives. What are you seeking? In the larger sense—beyond the motivation to earn a living, take care of your family, and meet other immediate needs—what are you striving to accomplish? Is the change you're contemplating consistent with that goal?

- What are the three most important accomplishments of your life to date? Consider the things you've accomplished in your family life and volunteer activities, as well as those related to your career. Why do you consider these to be your most important achievements? What do they indicate about your values, personality, and abilities?

- What is the legacy you would like to leave behind, not only in your career but in other areas of your life?

- Cognitive capabilities are only one measure of intelligence. Other capabilities include logical-mathematical, observational, scientific, musical, athletic, interpersonal, self-awareness, and written and verbal communications skills. Which of the various intelligences would you rate most highly in yourself? Which would you rate lowest?

- What do you see as your career options today? How likely are they to correspond with meeting your personal needs and fulfilling your goals? Compare the various options available to you according to these criteria.

- What obstacles do you confront in achieving your life's goals? What, if anything, have you done to overcome them? What obstacles still remain, and how do you plan to attack them?

Identifying Your Strengths

We all assume that there are some things we're particularly good at. But what exactly are those things? Could you define them precisely, and defend why you believe them to be so? Here's an exercise that will help you do just that.

Exercise: Analyzing and Understanding Your Accomplishments

Identify at least three specific accomplishments in your career or personal life. Write a brief description of each, including the following points:

- What was the situation? What was at stake? What obstacles stood in the way of success?
- What specific actions did you (or your team) take?
- What was the outcome of your action? How was it measured? What impact did it have?
- In what way was your contribution important to the outcome?

Once those three scenarios have been developed, patterns should emerge, since it is likely that you've called on certain skills—your major strengths—to achieve whatever successes you've achieved. Categorize those skills and list them. For example, you may find that you have certain:

- Intellectual skills: you're a problem solver, analytical, creative, practical, articulate.

Eyes Front

Let's be honest. Many physicians now in the market for opportunities outside clinical practice feel they're there because of circumstances beyond their control. Some are frustrated. Some are even angry. In an interview, however, let the future be the focus. What prospective employers want to hear about is what you can contribute to their prospects for success, not the grievances of the past. So if you've got an axe to grind, leave it at home.

- Interpersonal skills: you're a team player, dependable, good at directing others, persuasive, collaborative.
- Motivational skills: you're tenacious, highly energetic, determined, a self-starter, stimulated by challenge, good at handling stress.

In other words, what are the positive skills, behaviors, and qualities you demonstrate consistently?

Identifying Your Developmental Needs

None of us can do everything and do it well. Taking stock, you've identified your strengths. But that's only one part of the picture. We all have developmental needs as well.

Now, therefore, identify three situations whose outcomes you wish you could change. Describe them in writing, using the same outline as on page 13, except substitute for the last question (In what way was your contribution important to the outcome?) the following:

- What went wrong? What did you do—or fail to do—that contributed to the outcome?
- What did you learn from the experience?
- What strategies could have been employed to achieve a more successful outcome?
- What skills did you lack that might have made a difference?
- What, if anything, have you done since then to acquire those skills?
- If you encountered a similar situation today, would you be better prepared to handle it? Why?

Remember, nobody expects you to have been born knowing everything you need to know. Even our so-called failures are not failures when they inspire us to self-improvement. It's more important to be able to demonstrate openness to self-scrutiny and continual learning than it is to prove that we've never been wrong—and who would believe that contention, anyway?

20 Crucial Questions

Be prepared. The Boy Scouts long have recognized the wisdom of that motto. You should, too, as you contemplate running the interview gauntlet. Remember that the purpose of an interview is to get beyond the information that's already available to the interviewer from your resume or curriculum vitae. Interviewers want to know who you are, how you think, and how you react to the situation itself—and, given the brevity of the experience, they're going to make their judgments quickly. You can't afford to wait until the interview is under way to consider how your responses might affect those judgments.

Fortunately, you don't have to. Whatever the specific situation, most interviewers are likely to pose certain standard questions. While the questions themselves may be phrased in language that differs from interviewer to interviewer, most, after all, need to cover the same ground to get at the same insights.

Following is a list of the 20 questions interviewers are most likely to ask. In reviewing them, I'll identify the questions that are likely to be behind the question actually asked. I'll also try to provide some suggestions on what kind of information might constitute the most productive response.

Before you proceed to the list, however, please take heed of this important **warning:** there's an important difference between anticipating what you may be asked and rehearsing canned responses. An interview will be a test of your listening and interpersonal skills as much as any other abilities, and an experienced interviewer will recognize immediately when you're not genuinely involved in the process.

> **There's an important difference between anticipating what you may be asked and rehearsing canned responses.**

So review this list, think through appropriate responses, then relax and let it happen, remembering that how you respond in an interview is likely to be at least as important as what you say.

There's one more caveat to keep in mind. The frame of reference for many of the following questions is the business world, and many interviewers may also share that orientation. As a physician, you may think of your business experience as limited. But think again. Remember that as you make a career transition, interviewers will probably be most interested in your basic skills, abilities, and potential. Medical training and practice offer many experiences that parallel the demands of the business world. You can draw on experiences in that pool in framing your responses to such questions.

If you are asked a question that assumes experience that you lack, it is appropriate to acknowledge that lack and then to respond in a hypothetical mode, describing how you believe you would have responded to a given situation, or discussing how you did respond in a similar situation that occurred in another context, such as in the management of your practice.

1. What they may ask: "Tell me about yourself."

What they really want to know: How do you respond to pressure? How focused are you? How do you organize your thoughts? Often, an interviewer who asks this kind of broad, open-ended question is likely to be less interested in exactly what you say than in the way in which your response is organized.

Hints: Expect the question. Then prepare—and practice—a concise, chronologically ordered account of the significant events of your life, education, and career, focusing primarily on your career. Other aspects of your life, such as volunteer commitments, may be appropriate to mention, provided they offer insights into personal interests and values that may be relevant to your work. Whatever information you select to present, however, keep your comments brief (2 minutes at most). Rambling on beyond that amount of time risks losing the attention of the interviewer and challenging the interviewer's control of the interview process. And you'll probably have the opportunity to expand on the points you want to emphasize in response to other questions.

2. What they may ask: "Why are you contemplating a change at this time?"

What they really want to know: What factors are contributing to your interest in making a career change? What do they say about your long-term goals and values? There's another reason why interviewers frequently ask this question—to determine whether you've been terminated from your previous position. If so, they'll also want to know the circumstances of the termination and how you've responded to the event.

Hints: For the interviewee who is indeed positively motivated to make a change, framing an answer to this question is easy: articulate as clearly, concisely, and positively as you can what you look forward to accomplishing through a change at the present time. You'll want to emphasize what you're hoping to move to, rather than escape from, so if your reason for wishing to make a change is a reaction to a negative situation, consider carefully how to present your decision in as positive a light as possible.

In the event that a termination has taken place, honesty really is the best policy. Many terminations, of course, occur for reasons that have nothing to do with the performance of the person terminated. Even if that is not clearly the case, it's important to convey in your response confidence that you have carefully considered the events that led to the termination, have learned from the experience, and are ready to move on from it in a positive mode.

3. What they may ask: "What makes this opportunity attractive to you?"

What they really want to know: Have you done your homework? Do you fully understand the needs of the organization and the position? Is there a good match between those needs and your personal and professional objectives?

Hints: Do your research. Be sure you do have something to contribute to the organization. Then be prepared to identify where your potential contributions and the organization's perceived needs coincide.

> **Do your research. Be sure you do have something to contribute to the organization.**

4. What they may ask: "What do you want from your work that you haven't been getting?"

What they really want to know: How realistic are your expectations? How insightful are you in matching your expectations to your qualifications?

Hints: Every job has pluses and minuses, so the challenge is to delineate one or two realistic career objectives without resorting to the recitation of a gripe list.

A special word of warning: Never, under any circumstances, say anything that may be construed as critical of your current employer.

5. What they may ask: "What have been the most significant disappointments in your career?"

What they really want to know: How able are you to learn from experience and apply what you've learned to new challenges?

Hints: You can turn the apparent negatives in your career into positives by briefly relating one or two instances in which you would do things differently if you could do them over again, emphasizing what you learned from the experience and how you might relate it to the present opportunity.

6. What they may ask: "What are your major strengths?"

What they really want to know: What are the strengths you rely on for success? What particular skill sets have you called on—intellectual, interpersonal, organizational, etc—that have contributed to your success in situations you've encountered?

Hints: It's likely that you'd be able to list your strengths, but you need more than your own opinion to convince a potential employer that they exist. Be prepared with brief anecdotes that demonstrate how each of your strengths has contributed to successful outcomes in actual situations.

7. What they may ask: "What are your major developmental needs?"

What they really want to know: How insightful are you, and how open to self-analysis and self-improvement? How capable are you of identifying shortcomings and learning from mistakes?

Hints: Calling on the analysis you've made in preparing for the interview, identify those areas in which you plan to make improvements, then explain what you're planning to do about them.

8. What they may ask: "What are the most important business decisions you have made?"

What they really want to know: To what degree have your decision-making and risk-taking skills been tested? How did you pass the test?

Hints: Be sure you can offer two brief stories illustrating important professional decisions you have been called on to make, cogently summarizing the circumstances, what strategies you employed, and the outcome.

9. What they may ask: "What is the most complex business analysis you have had to make?"

What they really want to know: How keen are your analytic skills? To what degree have they been tested?

Bridging The Gap

In preparing for a job interview, you'll be focusing primarily on learning as much as you can about the type of business, particular organization, and individuals you'll encounter. In short, you'll be trying to understand as much as you can about the new world you're contemplating entering. But it's unrealistic to expect that your interviewer is undergoing a similar process to better understand the world you come from. It's your responsibility to bridge the understanding gap. You may see the relevance of your medical training and experience to a new career opportunity. But if those interviewing you lack knowledge of the medical world, they may not. A practical solution: Don't assume that your interviewer knows the medical environment. Do be prepared to explain fully how your background dovetails with the job requirements.

Hints: Again, you'll need to be prepared to cite a specific instance, this time one that illustrates how you've used business data to achieve a business objective.

10. What they may ask: "How do you choose members of your team?"

What they really want to know: Are you capable of analyzing a problem or situation and identifying the appropriate skills that will be required to address it? What attributes do you consider valuable in the business context?

Hints: Team building is essentially a test of problem-solving skills, so being able to articulate your rationale for team selection offers an interviewer affirmation of your analytic skills. In addition, what you expect of others may tell a lot about what can be expected of you. Be sure you've thoroughly thought through what personal and professional characteristics are appropriate for the environment, and why you think they are.

11. What they may ask: "How would you describe your management style?"

What they really want to know: Are you capable of amending your management style to adapt to different challenges?

Hints: Brief anecdotes that demonstrate how you've employed different approaches to addressing different situations can attest to desirable flexibility in your approach to problem solving.

12. What they may ask: "How do you influence others to buy into your ideas?"

What they really want to know: Are you capable of leadership?

Hints: Again, one or two real-life anecdotes provide the most vivid demonstration of ability.

13. What they may ask: "Under what circumstances have associates relied on you?"

What they really want to know: Have your leadership skills been tested? Under what circumstances? What was the outcome?

Hints: Collegiality is the essence of medicine. Even if you've never been officially designated a member or leader of a team, it is unlikely that you will be unable to identify experiences in your professional life in which you have worked in concert with others.

14. What they may ask: "Describe your relationships with your best and your worst bosses."

What they really want to know: How refined are your interpersonal and political skills?

Hints: Discussing your best relationship is easy. The challenge lies in responding to the latter part of the question. The iron-clad rule is: never, ever mention names. Let's say, though, that the interviewer might well be able to identify about whom you're speaking, on the basis of your background. Then the best response may be to diplomatically sidestep the issue. Acknowledge that you prefer not to speak specifically about someone on whom your comments might reflect negatively. Then frame a more generic response, relating, for example, the reasons why you experienced frustration or disappointment in a previous situation, such as not having been given as much responsibility as you felt prepared for.

> **The iron-clad rule is: never, ever mention names.**

15. What they may ask: "How has competition affected you, positively and negatively?"

What they really want to know: Are you a competitor? Do you perceive the stress of competition as a positive or a negative motivator?

Hints: This is an opportunity to demonstrate how you have functioned successfully, even under severe stress. Be realistic, however; everybody recognizes that stress has at least some negative consequences. Knowing how stress affects you and demonstrating how you have learned to manage its negative aspects is the test you must pass.

16. What they may ask: "Which of your accomplishments has been the source of the most satisfaction to you?"

What they really want to know: What motivates you?

Hints: Because the real purpose here is to gain insight into what makes you tick, be sure you can not only identify several accomplishments, but articulate why they're the source of special satisfaction to you.

17. What they may ask: "What were the most difficult political decisions you have had to make?"

What they really want to know: How politically astute are you?

Hints: Consider your successes. Which involved risks, sensitivities, or other political nuances? What factors did you weigh in developing a strategy to address them? You should be able to succinctly summarize the situation, the political implications, and your solution.

18. What they may ask: "What is the most intellectually challenging thing you have ever done?"

What they really want to know: What kinds of problems do you like to solve? How capable are you of learning and applying knowledge to new situations?

Hints: Review the challenges you have confronted which demonstrate your capabilities.

19. What they may ask: "What do you feel is essential to sustaining a successful business over the long run?"

What they really want to know: What is your business philosophy? What are your business values?

Hints: Again, researching the prospective employer and understanding the organization's strengths and weaknesses is essential to framing a good response, especially one that will permit you to link the contribution you could make to the organization's needs and goals.

20. What they may ask: "How do you define personal success?"

What they really want to know: What are your personal values? Are they in harmony with your business philosophy, and theirs?

Hints: Be honest. Remember that, in the last analysis, you want not only to land a job, but to land the job that's right for you. If the opportunity at hand does not offer what you need to ultimately achieve personal success, it's better to find out at the time of the interview than after spending years on the job.

> **Be honest. Remember that, in the last analysis, you want not only to land a job, but to land the job that's right for you.**

Setting the Stage

One of the most important objectives of a job interview is to establish a relationship between the interviewer and you. The task is not necessarily an easy one. You have only a short time in which to accomplish the objective. Your partner in the process—the interviewer—has an agenda that may differ from yours. Your control of the process will not be total, to say the least (although you do, through your responses to questions and the questions you ask, retain some measure of control).

Remember, though, that your goal throughout the process is not to take charge of the other participant, to win a confrontation, or to make instant decisions. Rather, your goal should be to set the stage for an exchange—to present yourself in such a way that your partner will be able to see that you could potentially be a member of his or her team, that you have the skills and experience that the organization needs, and that your personality and values mesh with those of others in the organization.

You Are What You Wear

Clothes may not really make the man—or woman—but they say a lot about us even before we open our mouths. The corporate culture of most organizations tends to dictate an unspoken dress code (and some may even have one that's written). Looking like you belong sends a subtle message about how you might fit in. So thinking about how you look and what to wear to the interview is not as superficial a concern as some might believe.

As a general rule, it's safe to say that, when it comes to dress, it's best to err on the conservative side. For men and women alike, suits should be in conservative colors (blue or gray), and the style is best determined by walking through a Brooks Brothers shop or that of some other clothing retailer known to cater to the business person. If you haven't purchased a suit for this purpose for a while, an investment at this time may be in order. Put your trust in a good salesperson for a reliable clothier; explain the reason for your purchase, and he or she is likely to be able to guide you in making an appropriate choice.

If time permits, walking or driving by the organization before the day of your interview will give you a chance to observe what employees are wearing and provide some insight into what might be appropriate apparel.

The Unspoken Clues

Body language tells a lot about us, too. A whole social science has developed around how we communicate nonverbally, and as trial lawyers, those who train interviewers, and others who use videotaped personal interaction as a tool know, when two people are really communicating, their bodies will unconsciously fall into a kind of dance of complementary motions. Although it is far beyond the purview of this booklet to delve into all the meaning and nuances of that dance, here are some tips about the signals we subconsciously send.

- Maintain eye contact—it signals confidence. Too much eye contact may signal aggression, however, while too little may signal lack of confidence or some other negative emotional content. Maintaining eye contact approximately 70% of the time is considered to be just about the right amount.

- Our bodies speak even when we are silent. A fixed body position may indicate aggression or amazement, folded arms could signal withdrawal or uncertainty, while a body turned slightly away from a listener

Two Strikes that Can Put You Out of the Game

To get the job, you have to have the opportunity for an interview. But some qualified physicians never even get that far in the process. Why? One recruiter experienced in placing physicians in management positions points out a couple of all too common failings that may count a physician out before he or she ever gets in the game.

Poor telephone skills. Long before you have the opportunity to meet face to face with an interviewer and put the strategies outlined in this document into practice, it's likely that you'll have a first encounter with the representative of a prospective employer via telephone. Making the cut requires the ability to articulate succinctly, but saliently, the reason why you're interested in and may be qualified for a job. Because medical training rarely includes instruction in verbal communication skills, many physicians fail this initial test.

Failure to accommodate basic business etiquette. Among mature physicians especially, the lack of certain basic business tools, such as the ability to use word processing equipment is endemic. That note you scrawl out by hand or the CV that doesn't conform to the rules of good resume writing, may, in your view, be adequate to serve its purpose. But your lack of conformance to the niceties of basic business etiquette may signal an inability or unwillingness to adapt to a new environment, a much larger issue in the eyes of a recruiter.

Different Folks, Different Strokes—Learning the Unspoken Language of Business

Few physicians are trained in the nuances of appropriate business etiquette. So it's not surprising that some may be ill prepared to present themselves in a manner that is likely to convince a potential employer of their credibility as a businessperson. Further complicating matters is that much miscommunication arises not as a result of the spoken word, but from the messages we subliminally send each other in the more subtle ways in which we communicate. Consider these scenarios.

- You're scheduling an interview. Your schedule is tight, especially these days when efficient time management is more important than ever before. So you suggest an early morning or late evening meeting, or somehow try to work the interview in between seeing patients. What's wrong with this picture? Although your time is valuable, the interviewer may resent the suggestion that it's more important than his or hers. Business meetings should be scheduled during regular business hours. If that means taking time from your practice, consider it an investment in the future.

- A midday meeting is set, but, still, time is short. To save as much of it as possible, you dash across town from the office or hospital without stopping to change from your usual workday garb. What's wrong? A white coat and stethoscope are important symbols in the health care setting, commanding respect. In the business environment, appearing that way may send a different message: that you're out of your depth or belong in a different league. Failure to appear in appropriate business attire may say something about you before you have a chance to utter a word.

- You're undergoing an interview. Time is limited, so you want to make every moment count. Used to taking charge, you use the time to cram in as much information about yourself as possible. What's wrong? While taking charge can be an admirable characteristic in some settings and under some circumstances, it's important not to seem to seize control from an interviewer during a job interview. What's more, the interview should be a dialogue and not a monologue. Your role is not just to sell yourself, but to gather information and demonstrate interest about the opportunity being presented. Failure to do so can be interpreted as lack of sufficient interest, or even arrogance on your part.

Adapted, with permission, from *Medical Practices & Managed Care* (Chicago, Ill: American Medical Association; 1995).

may indicate boredom. To communicate openness, maintain an upright body posture, edging forward slightly, with your hands in a comfortable position.

- Your smile is important. Use it often, because the interviewer is likely to reflect it.
- A vocal monotone may create boredom, and a fading tone signals an unconscious desire to leave. However, fluctuations in tone can keep a listener listening. Modulate your voice accordingly.
- Gestures can either be distracting or encourage listening. Nodding signals that we are involved, listening actively, and eager to hear more. Open arms are another indicator of willingness to receive more. Other kinds of gestures —demonstrating an all-encompassing look at the market by shaping the space in front of you as though you hands were moving along the circumference of a large ball, for example—may help illustrate a story, but unless you are a skilled presenter, select those you use with care.

Active Listening

We can also demonstrate our receptiveness through active listening. Listening actively takes energy and commitment and may be a challenge, especially to those who have experienced numerous interviews, which, after a time, may all seem to cover the same ground. Here are some of the characteristics that distinguish active from passive listening.

Passive Listeners	Active Listeners
Are inattentive	Are alert to all levels of meaning
Criticize the delivery	Respond to content
Look for argument	Respond when the message is understood
Listen for facts only	Look for central themes
Take too many notes	Write down key points only
Are easily distracted	Expend energy being attentive
Display emotion at "trigger" words	Keep an open mind
Make statements	Summarize, respond to nonverbal cues, use open-ended questions

Taking Notes

Whether to take notes during an interview is a decision that requires judgment on your part. Note taking can be distracting, especially in early stages of an interview. However, it's likely that some period of time may elapse between an initial interview and subsequent follow-up interviews, and it is risky to rely entirely on memory to retain important information during that interval. Therefore, it's important to find a quiet place immediately after an interview and record whatever important information you wish to retain.

If you do choose to take notes during the interview itself, that process should occur later in the interview as more complex information is shared with you. One way to solve the dilemma is to wait until data or other detailed material is discussed, then ask whether taking notes would be too distracting. In that way you have signaled the seriousness of your intent to understand that information presented to you without risking seeming insensitive to the potentially intrusive nature of note taking. However you approach the subject, keep in mind the importance of active listening.

A Question of Attitude

It may not be fair, but perception can be more real than reality when it comes to impressing a prospective employer. Unfortunately, many laypersons have the preconceived notion that doctors can be an arrogant lot. So, behaviors that seem innocent enough to you may be open to misinterpretation by others.

Consider the real-life case of the physician who was being considered for a job in industry. Three interviews, all to be conducted in quasi-social settings, were arranged. In each instance, the physician kept the representative of the company sent to escort him to the event waiting for exactly 10 minutes. What's 10 minutes in the larger scheme of things? Just enough to confirm a preconception that physicians are arrogant and thus likely to be poor team players. Not surprisingly, the physician never got the job.

Think that's unfair? Consider this: you can even be misjudged by behaviors that aren't your own. In some settings, special stature comes with being the spouse of a physician. If your spouse is to be involved in the interview process, be sure he or she shares your understanding of the importance of monitoring words and deeds so as not to reinforce any unfortunate misconceptions about physicians held by those you'll be meeting.

Running the Gauntlet

The moment of truth has arrived. You've done your homework, researched the opportunity, thought through responses to the questions you're most likely to be asked, and armed yourself with insight into the cues of unspoken communication. Now let's see what the actual interview will involve.

No interview will adhere neatly to an established pattern. Each, however, represents a process in which certain things are likely to occur. You can't control the interview—that remains the domain of the interviewer. But you can try to ensure that you complete each essential part of the interview process in a way that avoids obvious mistakes, enhances your attractiveness as a candidate, and provides you with the information you will need to make your own decision about the opportunity, should it eventually be offered to you.

Opening Moves

At the beginning of the interview, both parties will probably be focused on establishing rapport and putting the other party at ease. This may be accomplished by means of small talk about the weather, the location, sports, family, entertainment, or current events. Although the subject of discussion at this point may be trivial, the interlude itself is important, since it will create that all-important first impression of you. Therefore, be sure your comments, whatever the subject, are positive, upbeat, and energetic. Negativism, whatever the context, is likely to color the interviewer's memory, even though the actual content of your comments may soon be forgotten.

If you are given the opportunity to choose the subject, be sure to avoid any that might be viewed as political or carry some other form of emotional baggage with them. One possible way in which to find a positive subject is to survey the interviewer's office for something that may provide an opportunity for comment. For example, a lawyer, interviewing with a law firm, commented on the beautiful view of a lake that could be seen from the interviewer's office window. That led the lawyer naturally to mention that, as a runner, he ran past the building each day. Although he had not previously known it, he learned that the interviewer had been a sprinter in college, a fact that created instant rapport and set a positive tone for the subsequent exchange of information.

That important first impression will be shaped by more than words. The handshake you offer will also leave a lasting impression. The hand should be dry (damp palms can be controlled by leaving your palms open to the air while waiting to meet the interviewer) and the handshake firm, among both men and women, consisting of a quick motion up and down that is repeated two or three times. Smiling and making eye contact during the handshake reinforces the openness of the gesture.

Exchanging Information—The Heart of the Process

But the most essential task you must undertake is to ensure that the interview itself consists of a good exchange of information—an exchange that will demonstrate to the interviewer how your skills and experience match the needs of the organization, and one that will elicit the information you need to assess whether the opportunity is the right one for you. Your task may be complicated by a problem that is all too common, if not often acknowledged—the fact that, despite the importance of selecting team members as a function of management, a surprising number of managers are untrained in the interview process. For that reason, you may need to take an active, if subtle, role in keeping the process moving in the right direction.

There is a delicate balance to achieve, however. Ask most interviewers their reaction immediately after conducting an interview and the response is likely to be something in this vein: "I had a good feeling about her" or "I don't know; something just didn't feel right about him." Rational or not, the fact of the matter is that, however diligent the interviewer is in objectively gathering information, the most important response to the interviewee is the subjective one.

So, while pursuing your personal objectives of gathering the information you want and providing the information you believe the interviewer needs to appreciate your qualifications, keep in mind the importance of not seeming to wrest control of the situation from the person who should be in charge—the interviewer. In the last analysis, most interviewers' decisions depend more on whether they liked and were comfortable with the interviewee than on any of the information presented. To ensure your interviewer's comfort level, remember that the interview should be an arena for an exchange of information—and not a combat zone from which to emerge victorious. Here are some hints that may help.

> **Remember that the interview should be an arena for an exchange of information—and not a combat zone from which to emerge victorious.**

- Answer each question honestly and fully, but try to limit each response to no more than 2 or 3 minutes in length.

- The interviewer's task will be to determine whether your skills and experience match the needs of the position; yours will be to demonstrate that you are capable of achieving success in the kind of situation the position represents. Remember, though, that your experiences need not exactly duplicate those required by the position in order to be relevant. Verbal cues like the following may be helpful: "The position you've described is very similar to what I did at...," "That situation is similar to the one I encountered when...," "That reminds me of something that we tackled successfully at...."

- Since it is as important to you to gather information as it is to give it during the interview, whenever appropriate, consider completing your responses with a question or a statement that might elicit the information you seek. Let's say, for example, that you've been asked to describe a problem you've encountered. Having done so, you could conclude your description with a comment of this nature: "From what you've told me so far, the department in which this position is located seems to be facing a similar challenge. Could you tell me more about that?" A caveat, however: be judicious in using this approach so as not to leave the interviewer with the impression that you are trying to avoid or deflect his or her line of questioning.

- Be alert to the possibility that an interviewer may seem to overlook or not fully understand something about your skills or background that may be relevant to your qualifications. When that occurs, it's not inappropriate to ask interviewers if it would be useful to know more about X, Y, or Z. That's one way you can try to ensure that really essential information is not lost in the interview process.

Coming to Closure

Each interview has its own rhythm, and you will probably sense when an interview is coming to a close. When all the essential questions have been asked and answered, that's the time to reiterate your interest in the opportunity and verify that you are still considered a viable candidate. Here are some approaches that might be appropriate:

> *"I have learned a lot about the organization and what is needed. Thank you. I must say that I am very interested in learning more. I have the sense that my experience and my style fit here. I would be very interested in taking the next steps. Do you see anything that might prevent that at this point?"* This is a very bold and direct approach. Some interviewers may find it difficult to answer the question directly; others will not.

> *"I am very excited about what your organization is attempting to do. I think the market needs it. I believe that your strategy is pointed in the right direction. I could see myself making contributions in a number of ways. After having spent some time together, is there anything you might suggest that I can do to demonstrate more effectively my interest in or skills related to this opportunity?"* A subtler approach to achieving the same objective, this is a question most interviewers will be more comfortable responding to.

> *"I like what I hear about the organization, what it stands for, how it operates, the talent it represents. Before we part today, could you summarize for me the two or three things that will be absolutely required for someone like myself to be successful in this position? I just want to be sure that we haven't missed exploring my qualifications thoroughly."* This represents perhaps the

subtlest approach of all, one that leaves the summing up to the discretion of the interviewer, but still provides you with the opportunity to clarify points or fill in gaps if the interviewer appears not to have perceived all of the relevant qualifications that you wish to point out.

No interview should conclude without you knowing what to expect next. Some interviewers will offer that information; others will not. If the next steps in the selection process are not discussed, be sure to ask: "What are the next steps?" "Where do we go from here?" or "What can you tell me about the next steps in your selection process?"

Following Up—Two Important Exercises

Exercise 1

Few significant positions are filled as the result of just one interview. Recapping in writing the information that you have gathered in each interview is extremely important, therefore, in helping you be sure that you have all the information you need. Generate a simple checklist that can be used to determine whether you have all the information you need, while identifying any gaps that you may wish to fill in the next round.

Exercise 2

Every interview you participate in should be followed up immediately with a letter to every person who has interviewed you, briefly thanking the interviewer for his or her time and interest and reiterating the major reasons why you believe you are qualified for the position. One way in which to emphasize your interest in the position is to make a mental note, during the interview, of any issue that seems to be of particular concern or interest to the interviewer. Making reference to that matter in your follow-up letter will demonstrate the degree to which you were attentive during the interview and reinforce your commitment to making a contribution to the position.

Special Situation

Some interview situations will involve being interviewed by a group of interviewers. When confronted with such an event, try to learn in advance the names and titles of those who will be participating. The research on the organization that you have already done should be reviewed to ensure that you have an understanding of the roles played by those with whom you will be meeting.

Group interviews may be formal or informal proceedings. As introductions are made, listen for clues as to the climate in which the interview will be conducted, and adjust your responses accordingly. Although remembering names is always important in the business and professional world, it is especially important in such a proceeding. Therefore, be sure you can identify who's who among your interviewers, and always refer to each person by name—and title, if appropriate—when directly addressing them.

Relationship building—that process of attempting to find a common personal ground with the interviewer—is more complicated, but no less important, in a group interview. That period of time while the participants are assembling and before the formal part of the meeting has begun is the best time to try to establish that rapport.

Be sure you can identify who's who among your interviewers.

It is not uncommon for group interviews to occur over lunch or dinner. Prospective employers may also wish to ascertain whether any personal obstacles to a successful transition into the position may exist, especially where relocation or other lifestyle changes may be involved. Recognizing the importance of spousal support as an ingredient in professional success, an organization seeking to fill a position may also invite a spouse to participate in the interview. When that occurs, the spouse needs to be prepared for the encounter by being thoroughly briefed on the nature of the organization and the opportunity, your degree of interest in it, and the positions and backgrounds of the participants. Any possible concerns on the part of the spouse should be identified and, it is hoped, resolved, before the meeting.

Like one-on-one interviews, group interviews should be followed up with personalized letters to each interviewer. The same rules apply: thank the interviewer for his or her time, summarize the points that sell your candidacy, and, when possible, attempt to add to the letter a comment that demonstrates that you have brought away from the interview insight into issues of particular concern to the interviewer.

A Final Word

Some time ago, a candidate for a high-level position with a major oil company traveled to the West Coast to be personally interviewed by the company's chief executive officer. The CEO had one question, and one question only, and gave the candidate exactly 10 minutes of his time in which to answer. The question: "Why should I hire you?"

I can't tell you how the candidate answered. It can only be hoped that he'd done his homework on the organization, the position in question, and the personality of the CEO, as well as the essential self-assessment that might have contributed to formulating an appropriate response.

> **"Why should I hire you?"**

In the previous pages, we've laid out a process by which to prepare for an interview. We've described in a neat, orderly fashion the scenario by which the interview process is supposed to be conducted. Now we have a confession to make: unfortunately, real life rarely follows the course it's supposed to.

If that truth is somewhat disconcerting, take heart. While I can't promise you that the interaction that occurs in the interview process will neatly follow the script presented here, we can assure you that if you've prepared yourself according to the process that's been outlined, you should be prepared to deal deftly with whatever actual events occur.